I0759347

Could It Be Gluten?

A guide to understanding the facts about the gluten free diet.

by EM KENNEDY

The cover, interior content, and GFEM logo are all
property of Em Kennedy.

Copyright © 2021

Emily May Kennedy

All rights reserved

ISBN: 9781799219897

COULD IT BE GLUTEN?

In this book, we will discuss the reasons and method of going gluten free. There is a lot of controversy on this subject and I hope that this guide will help clear up a lot of fiction and replace it with facts.—EM KENNEDY

A. What is gluten sensitivity?

    a. Diagnosing celiac disease

    b. Learning the symptoms of gluten sensitivity

    c. What else could it be?

B. What are the chances I have of developing gluten sensitivity?

    a. The different levels of gluten sensitivity

    b. The other foods that could be at the root of

the problem

    c. Is it allergies?

C. What do I do now that I suspect gluten sensitivity?

    a. Get tested

    b. Start keeping a food diary consistently and accurately

    c. Embark on the elimination diet

D. How do you go gluten free?

    a. Starting in the kitchen with foods

    b. Cosmetics

    c. Shampoo

    d. Deodorant

    e. Soaps

A. WHAT IS GLUTEN SENSITIVITY?

a. What exactly is gluten sensitivity? This question is a hard one to explain because of the *inconsistency of symptoms*. Everyone is different and his or her body may not react the same way as someone else's. In addition, learning the possible symptoms does not diagnose someone. **There are blood tests that can confirm or eliminate suspicion for Celiac disease, but gluten sensitivity can only be diagnosed through trial and error, or in other words, <u>the elimination diet.</u>**

Gluten sensitivity is something that at one time was rarely heard of, but a few years ago it began emerging as more and more doctors became open to the fact that food allergies and sensitivities have a tremendous negative impact on one's health if left untreated. As this knowledge spread, more and more people had the gluten free diet recommended to them by healthcare professionals as an alternative to many other more invasive procedures like gallbladder surgery, weight loss surgery, or in some instances dependence on steroid, or pain drugs, etc.

The first bit of advice I will give is something I learned the hard way: ***Do not start a gluten free diet until Celiac disease is ruled out!*** If you are very sick tell the doctor when you call to get an appointment, but do not change anything just yet. They will more than likely send you for an upper endoscopy (upper GI), this is a simple, virtually pain free procedure that allows the doctor to take a sample of your small intestine to look for gluten damage caused by Celiac disease. <u>You have to be eating wheat for at least six weeks beforehand for the biopsy of your small intestine to be accurate.</u> They will not diagnose Celiac disease unless <u>severe</u> damage is present. This test is very important; please do not decline to have it done just because someone else told you how bad it was for him or her. I personally have had it done several times and feel that it is just as simple as getting dental work. You will fast the night before. Then when it's time they will sedate you and insert a small tube down your throat with a camera so they can take pictures of your esophagus, stomach, and small intestine. They also can take a biopsy (a small tissue sample) for testing under a microscope. That is how they look for damage to the small intestine caused by Celiac disease.

b. Secondly, **learn the symptoms.** The symptoms of gluten sensitivity are much like the symptoms of Celiac disease. Telling the two apart can be difficult. <u>That is why it is highly recommended that a Celiac test be done first.</u> If you do go gluten free and the symptoms disappear, they still will not diagnose you unless a positive biopsy had been taken.

Celiac disease symptoms include but are not limited to:

Diarrhea that is foul smelling and fatty

Lactose intolerance

Weight loss in spite of high calorie intake

Severe abdominal pain (especially after meals)

Irritable bowel syndrome

Bloating

Iron deficiency

Unexplainable fatigue

GERD that does not respond well to treatment (having to take medicine for it long term)

Vitamin deficiencies

Gluten sensitivity symptoms:

Diarrhea

Constipation (usually goes back and forth between the two)

Lactose intolerance

Weight loss or weight gain in drastic amounts

(For me it could be a loss of up to 10 pounds in a week!)

Abdominal pain and discomfort continually

Bloating

Needing to take multivitamins continually, but not really experiencing the benefit from them.

Severe PMS

Fatigue

Mind fogginess

Acid reflux and vomiting

Hypoglycemia (Feeling like you are going to lose it if you do not eat and having pass out spells from low blood sugar.)

Diabetic like symptoms (low/high or fluctuating blood sugar)

Addiction and love for foods containing wheat, barley, oats, or rye (bread, sweets, etc.)

Always finding yourself in the kitchen looking for something to eat to help your stomach calm down

Vivid dreams

Constant dry mouth

Rash on the skin around the mouth

Teeth grinding

Progressive decrease in eyesight particularly night vision

Pregnancy complications and discomfort above normal

Preterm delivery

Painful and prolonged labor

Small underweight babies

Colic

Constant spitting up

Stunted growth in children

Delayed puberty in teens

Lack of menstrual cycle

Eczema

Asthma

Autoimmune diseases

Constant croup like attacks in young children

Decreased immune system (catching every bug that comes along)

These of course are just some of the most predominant symptoms of gluten sensitivity. You should never diagnose yourself based on symptoms alone because many illnesses have the same symptoms and something more serious could be underlying the problem. It requires some further looking into by a qualified physician (not every physician fits the bill; do not hesitate to get a second, or even third opinion).

c. The other possible illnesses that share some of the same symptoms of gluten sensitivity are:

Autoimmune thyroiditis

Hyperthyroidism

Hypothyroidism

Delayed reaction food allergies

Hormone imbalances

Sleep apnea related GERD

Ovarian cysts

Crohn's disease

Diverticulitis

Fibromyalgia

Malnutrition

Vitamin deficiency

Intestinal parasites

This of course, is not a complete list, merely a few of the more prevalent illnesses that have the same or similar symptoms as gluten sensitivity. It is up to your doctor to weigh out the facts and see whether testing is necessary. Remember it is always a long shot when going off symptoms alone.

B. WHAT ARE THE CHANCES I HAVE OF DEVELOPING GLUTEN SENSITIVITY?

a. ***There is always a chance that someone of any age will develop an allergy or intolerance even when none was present before.*** Mainly because of our imbalanced diets: we tend to eat the same things over and over again, not realizing that there is more to life than fast food or processed foods to pop in the microwave. These quick meals tend to be loaded with preservatives that in themselves take a toll on our health. In almost every fast food item or processed food, you will find wheat or gluten of some type. (Many fast food venues have started to offer "gluten free foods" as part of their menu, but when prepared on the same equipment, or in some cases fried in the very same oil as something containing wheat, they are not truly gluten free.) This wheat tends to be genetically modified to make the proteins stronger and easier to use, also making it harder to digest. The average person gets wheat in every meal of the day including snacks! Wheat is hard to digest because of its complex proteins, the main one being gluten. The average person's stomach and immune system is bombarded by this antagonist and does not get a break from it, not even for a day! No wonder their health is falling apart. When you constantly expose your immune system to an antagonist, your body will either get used to it, or start reacting to it. The result of this reaction is the unpleasant symptoms you are experiencing. It is just a matter of taking proper care of your body by giving it the nutrition it needs and the diversity of foods necessary for good health. If you knew that smoking caused cancer, would you smoke anyway? If you knew that drinking alcohol caused liver disease, wouldn't you avoid it? Just as we would avoid more obvious toxins that are precarious to our health, someone with a gluten sensitivity or Celiac disease should avoid gluten.

Someone could be slightly gluten intolerant and have symptoms like gas, bloating, and acid reflux. In this kind of situation, limiting your exposure down to only once a day at the most is good treatment to relieve symptoms. Also taking a high quality digestive enzyme and probiotics will also help.

Then there is a more severe intolerance called gluten sensitivity which causes more intense cramps, nausea, vomiting, diarrhea, passing out spells, and malnutrition to name a few of the symptoms; in this kind of situation complete avoidance to the protein gluten is the only way to relieve symptoms.

In addition, there is the worst possible gluten intolerance; this you find in Celiac Disease where the slightest bit of gluten does intestinal damage on top of all the side effects found in gluten sensitivity. In this kind of situation, complete avoidance of the protein gluten is the ONLY way to keep the disease from progressing.

b. Of course, gluten is not the only kind of food that plays an antagonistic roll; *there are several different foods that have similar ways of provoking the immune system into making you feel bad*. One of these is corn. Like wheat, corn is widely used and tends to be genetically modified. Corn can be found in most medications as the starch used to bind the medication together. (This may also be wheat, always check with the manufacturer to be sure). A corn intolerance is generally stemmed from a delayed reaction allergy to corn. **An allergy can cause you to have a feel good high as soon as you eat the problematic food by raising your blood pressure, and then crash you into exhaustion when the blood pressure drop hits later.**

Other than corn and wheat, there are other foods like meats and nuts, dairy and soy products. Some people even have intolerances to some fruits and vegetables causing them a wide range of health problems. _Any type of food that is eaten in excess and extremely often can become a problem._ Some people experience problems with several different foods at the same time, but mostly in a mild way.

c. Patch testing can be done to determine whether a delayed allergic reaction (or IgG reaction) is present. A delayed reaction carries with it several different symptoms but the most common one is a hay fever type of reaction, which shows up 48 to 72 hours after the initial exposure. _**A certified**_

<u>allergist should test someone who has a problem with chronic sinuses.</u> It is inexpensive and requires little discomfort compared to the wide range of benefits found in knowing what your allergies are.

Anyone who experiences an IgE antibody allergic reaction, such as swelling of the face, tongue, or throat should go to the emergency room immediately!

These kinds of reactions are not to be played around with or loss of life may occur. Do not ignore a severe allergic reaction, next time it happens it will be worse and could <u>kill</u> you! Get the help of a certified allergist to determine the underlying problem. EACH TIME YOU ARE EXPOSED TO AN ALLERGEN YOUR BODY PRODUCES MORE HISTAMINE

THUS MAKING A WORSE REACTION! <u>DO NOT RISK YOUR LIFE OR THE LIFE OF A LOVED ONE. GET TESTED!</u>

A lot of babies and young children have food allergies that their parents do not recognize. The parents generally suspect a so-called harmless intolerance like lactose intolerance, never realizing the seriousness of the problem. If your child suffers from chronic ear infections, colic, diarrhea, a rash on their bottom that will not clear up, or constant spitting up, get them tested for food allergies. Also be aware of the signs of a possibly serious food allergy. How does a child usually describe such symptoms?

I have an itchy mouth.

My tongue hurts.

I think I have a piece of hair stuck in my throat.

My neck hurts. (Placing their hands near their throat.)

I'm too tired to play. (If directly after a meal your child gets lethargic, you need to consider the possibility of a food allergy!)

My belly hurts.

My head hurts.

All of these and many more could be their way of telling you they are experiencing an allergic reaction. You, as the parent, know your child better than anyone else (especially if you are a stay at home mom). You need to observe your child to see if there is a possible correlation with the symptoms they have and the food they eat. If an allergy is suspected, do yourself and them a favor….Get Them Tested!

For those mothers who breastfeed: milk proteins, wheat proteins and several other complex food proteins are passed through breast milk to the baby. So yes, a baby who has never had solid foods can be experiencing gluten sensitivity if the mother eats wheat. Always be on the safe side and get tested if there is a possibility of gluten sensitivity or an allergy.

C. WHAT DO I DO NOW THAT I SUSPECT GLUTEN SENSITIVITY?

a. The first thing to do is, as I have already said, *GET TESTED.* Go to your doctor, tell them that you suspect gluten sensitivity, explain to them the symptoms you are experiencing, and ask them if they can test you. Usually your primary care physician will send you to an allergist and a *gastroenterologist.* These two types of specialist can perform the test necessary to check for food allergies and Celiac disease respectively. Once these are ruled out then it is up to you to determine how much you are willing to take before you head out on your own to discover the real problem. *No one knows your body the way you do.* If you have been suffering with these different symptoms for years and have spent thousands of dollars on doctors and specialist just to find that they tell you nothing is wrong, then this is definitely a turning point. *Many people are even told that it is all in their mind and are handed anxiety drugs, which do not help, simply because the doctors they are working with are not knowledgeable in the crucial area of gluten sensitivity or intolerance.* The choice is yours, keep spending money on drugs that cover up the symptoms without treating the problem, or set out on your own to find the real problem. *Someone who feels seriously bad all the time has an underlying condition, and it is not in their mind, it is real!*

b. *The second thing to do is to begin keeping an accurate food diary.* Make sure that you list all the different foods that you have eaten in the day. Serving size is of little importance unless you are counting calories, *but the different <u>ingredients </u>in the food are of <u>high importance.</u>* For example, you ate a biscuit at Hardees for breakfast, they do not list all the ingredients but you know that there is wheat, egg, pork (if it was bacon or sausage), and dairy (from the buttermilk and butter used to make the biscuits and the cheese), maybe even soy (a lot of cheese products contain soy). All these separate ingredients should be listed next to the name of the food (example: bacon, egg, and cheese biscuit). Also, list your symptoms. If you experience them right after or during eating a certain food, list it near that food. Once you have been doing this for a little while, look to see if there are any connections between what you are eating and how you are feeling. For instance, you ate that biscuit for breakfast, you did not feel any different, but at lunch, you ate a sub sandwich and felt sick afterward. This could be that it took a while for breakfast to make its way into your intestines to make you feel bad or it could be that you were having wheat again. It could also have been just another ingredient present in the sub and not the wheat at all!

The next page contains an example of a food diary entry, and the different foods associated with the symptoms:

Friday, November 9th 2016

Breakfast:

Bowl of cream of wheat, sugar, butter (wheat, dairy)

Glass of apple juice

Lunch:

Leftover spaghetti (wheat, from the noodles, tomato, hamburger, onions, peppers, garlic, from the sauce)

Glass of tea

Snack:

Almond joy (almond, coconut, soy, corn, dairy)

Pepsi cola (corn)

Donut (wheat, corn, dairy, soy)

Supper:

Bowl of big butter beans (beans, pork from the seasoning meat)

Biscuit with butter (wheat, soy, dairy)

Symptoms:

Felt really fatigued again today. I tried to eat healthy but still don't have any energy. Stomach cramped bad after supper again tonight. Mind is very foggy.

==Notice how with each meal, wheat was eaten!==

This looks like someone who really is trying to eat healthy, with what seems like a wide variety of foods. However, with a closer look provided by the food diary, you will see that wheat was present in some form in each meal of the day. *There are so many details involved in the way we eat that a food diary is the only way to remember and keep track of how often we eat a certain food.* You cannot accurately find out what is making you sick unless you know exactly what you are eating. Be sure to read labels and list every obvious ingredient. For example, dairy, wheat, soy, corn, peanuts, tree nuts (example: almonds), eggs, meat (example: beef), vegetables (example: carrots or cabbage), and spices (example: added spices like paprika, or garlic, or annatto found in cheese). ***The more detail***

you give, the easier it will be to find what is making you feel bad.

d. *Thirdly, start an elimination diet beginning with the food that you suspect the most based on your food diary entrees.* In the previous example, it was wheat so we will use this. Go through your kitchen and eliminate all sources of wheat. *Do not throw them away just avoid them for at least a week, <u>preferably two weeks</u>.* If you notice any improvement at all, <u>*make a note of it in your food diary.*</u> Then add back in the suspected food and see how it affects you. If you start feeling bad again, make a special note of that food and eliminate it. Continue this process until you find that you are feeling significantly better. If your food diary does not pin point any one particular food, try starting with wheat, then corn, then dairy, then soy etc. <u>Wheat is usually the one at fault because it is so widely used and genetically modified, causing the already hard to digest complex protein gluten to become even harder to digest.</u> **When done correctly, the elimination diet can be the most successful form of diagnoses when food intolerances or allergies are at the root of the problem.** **You do not have to swell up and die immediately to have an allergy present in your body. The delayed and even some of the more mild IgE allergies can cause other symptoms that tear your health down piece by piece.**

C. HOW DO YOU GO GLUTEN FREE?

The last section of this book has to deal strictly with going gluten free. *If you felt better when eliminating wheat through the elimination diet, try going gluten free.* Usually the protein at the root of the problem is the protein gluten. Eliminating gluten from your diet can take away the symptoms you are experiencing from a gluten sensitivity. Only when done *completely* can it yield such amazing results as disappearing fatigue, vanishing diarrhea, and eczema clearing up after years of itching and burning.

When I chose to go gluten free, I noticed after about a month that I had regained most of my night vision, which had gotten so bad I was falling while going to the bathroom at night. (Even with a nightlight on!) I also regained some of the muscle mass that had wasted away and regained strength that I had not experienced since a young teenage girl! I was able to tolerate heat better, and was not always flushed. My bowels straightened out in about two weeks and my GERD was gone immediately!!! My son's diarrhea that he had from birth left within a few days of going gluten free, and the rash on his bottom that had been there for years vanished! My youngest son who was just an infant at the time, lost his colicky ways, and stopped waking me up every few hours with sleep apnea that stopped his breathing! I no longer had to check to see if he was breathing because the reflux that was causing the apnea was gone taking the sleep apnea away with it! My eldest son had constipation almost continuously his whole life, and bad eczema particularly on his legs. He also had asthma that he had been taking medicine to control, and lethargy. All these left when we went gluten free!

Less sinus infections, less headaches, less mood swings, etc. I could go on and on but the results speak for themselves. I have been gluten free for years now, and still don't regret my decision because of the life-changing benefits it brought. Going gluten free was the first step we took towards better health; avoidance of other known food allergies was the second. Our lives changed significantly for the better from both of these treatments. Prayer, avoidance of known food sensitivities and allergies, and Chiropractic care are the only things that we have tried over the years that have really made a lasting difference in the chronic health problems we have encountered. As a family, we are Gluten free, and we believe in the Creator who created our bodies to heal themselves naturally. We also have learned that sometimes there are things hindering us from healing, and we must get rid of those hindrances if we expect to improve. (Chiropractic carries this view and is a very effective treatment for those who experience digestive issues.)

The reason I am writing this book is so that someone else can benefit from the information I have worked so hard to find. I want you to try it for yourself and reap the amazing result in your home. Why put up with second-rate health? Why deal with those petty annoying problems you were told you inherited and are stuck with, like sinuses, asthma, eczema, fatigue? Just because your parents have put up with it all their lives does not mean *you cannot make a difference in your own life right now.* You have made the first step in reading this book, now go on, complete the steps, and get the results you have always wanted – a healthy body! TAKE CHARGE OF YOUR HEALTH AND BE A WINNER, GO GLUTEN FREE!

a. *When you go gluten free, always start in the kitchen.* Finding gluten in the kitchen is challenging, but once you get the hang of it, it will become like a second nature. The most obvious places to look are things containing grains. Bread, biscuits, pie crust, pasta, canned soups and sauces, breaded meat or vegetables, gravies, candy, ice cream cones, cakes and snack cakes, donuts, pretzels, cereal, muffins, etc. Even salad dressings can contain gluten! Gluten is found in more than just wheat products. Things containing wheat, barley, oats, or rye all contain gluten. Not to mention there are several different names for wheat like Atta, Bulgur, Couscous, Durum, Einkorn, Emmer, Enriched wheat, all-purpose/ and self-rising flour, whole wheat flour, Farina, Gluten, Graham flour, high gluten/protein flour, bread flour, Kamut, Seitan, Semolina, Spelt (dinkel, farro), Triticale (a cross between wheat and rye), Triticum aestivum, Wheat bran, wheat flour, wheat germ, wheat starch. Anything manufactured on the same equipment as wheat or any of its gluten containing counterparts will also have gluten in it. So be careful when you make your selection of foods to eat.

There are several words to keep your eye out for when reading labels; malt, starch, modified food starch, cereal grain, wheat germ, malt flavoring, processed on the same equipment as wheat products, maltadextrin, emulsifier, stabilizer, grain alcohol. **Wheat, Tricticum, Spelt, Oats, Bran, Farina, Malt, and Barley can also be found attached to longer words but it all means a source of gluten.** *Just because something is wheat free does not* *mean it is gluten free!* Be careful to look for the words gluten free or the gluten free sign (which looks like a wheat stalk with a line crossed through it). It should be somewhere on the packaging. If there is no source of grains, also be sure to see if it has been *processed on the same equipment as wheat products*! A few good examples of this is tomato sauce, frozen vegetables, candy bars, ice cream, cheese products, canned soups, processed vegetables, rice cereal, or corn cereal and even some dry beans and rice products. *Always read the label!*

Fresh fruits and vegetables are the best choice when it comes to food, along with fresh (not breaded) meat. When you cook them, try not to use any seasonings unless you have confirmed with the manufacturer that they are gluten free (some spices have emulsifiers that could mean gluten). Of course, raw vegies and fruits are great for you just how they are, especially if they are organic. Eating them in a salad, blending them into a smoothie, or chopping them into a salsa is a few ways you can use them raw.

Also, be sure to check all your medications for gluten. Pills need a starch to bind the medicine to and this could be gluten. Call the manufacturer to be sure. While going through your kitchen, also be sure to look through the refrigerator for mayonnaise, salad dressing, or other condiments that have gluten in them. (A big one most people miss is the opened jar of mayonnaise, peanut butter, jelly, or other condiment that has been used on bread containing wheat. When you spread peanut butter on a piece of bread, and then insert the knife back into the jar, you have just contaminated that jar with gluten. Yes, it is that big of a deal if you want to be completely gluten free. This is one that I struggled with when I first went gluten free, making myself sick many times before I realized it.) Check all labels. Even cheese products need to be checked. Drinks are a great hiding place for gluten, always read the labels. Do not hesitate to call the manufacturer, they are used to hearing it and may even have a gluten statement as part of their automated menu.

If you are a beginner then you should follow these steps carefully:

STEP 1: Go through the refrigerator and take out all the things that clearly list wheat or any words listed above that mean gluten. Call the manufacturer about the things you are unsure about.

STEP 2: Go through your cabinets for the non-perishable foods that have a source of gluten listed on the labels. Call the manufacturer for any products you are unsure of. BE EXTREMELY CAUTIOUS WITH PRODUCTS CONTAINING GRAINS SUCH AS BREAD, CEREAL AND PASTA. Almost always they mean a source of gluten. It doesn't mean you won't get to eat bread, cereal, or pasta anymore...it just means you will need to buy a gluten free form of these foods. There are so many products on the market these days that taste good and are good for you.

STEP 3: Check your spices and flavorings for gluten by calling the manufacturer.

STEP 4: Call the manufacturer about all drinks and medication that you are taking to look for gluten.

STEP 5: Relax and enjoy your gluten free kitchen! Treat yourself with a gluten free version of your favorite food. (For recipes, such as lasagna, brownies, chocolate chip cookies, apple cake, and homemade white bread visit www.glutenfreeEm.com!)

b. *Another place that most people forget to look is cosmetics.* If you use makeup, acne cream, or lotions, be sure to ask the manufacturer whether there is gluten present in the product or any of its ingredients. Some people say that it is overdone to include nonfood products in your gluten search, but if it comes in contact with your hands and then you touch something you eat, it will be in your system. Please do not ignore this important area when going gluten free.

c. *Shampoo is one of the most important nonfood items that should be careful checked for gluten.* I have read that hair follicles absorb gluten, and can make you as sick as if you had eaten a piece of gluten-filled bread. I have also read that it cannot, so I tested it myself. I went without my gluten containing shampoo for several weeks, and then went back to using it. I found that gluten containing shampoos and hair care products made me feel very ill the very same day! I have also found that they irritate my scalp and cause intense itching and even psoriasis. If you have gone gluten free but are still experiencing a small amount of fatigue, change your shampoo it could be the problem! A shampoo that is clearly labeled gluten free can be found at your nearby health food store, or pharmacy.

d. *Deodorant is another big place to look but not as important as shampoo.* If you are experiencing any kind of skin irritation from using your deodorant, call the manufacturer about it to be sure there is no gluten present in any of the ingredients. If you experience burning or itching after applying deodorant to your underarms there is a big chance it has gluten in it.

c. *Soap is often forgotten about, but can also be a source of gluten. Soft soaps are the main sources, so call the manufacturer!* When unsure, try to observe how your skin responds to it. If it makes you itch or a rash appears (even if it is delayed until you have used the soap continuously for a week or so), you can guarantee there is something in it you are sensitive to. Severe dry skin and eczema are often made worse by soaps that have a hidden source gluten in them. If it makes you flare up, avoid it.

These are the few simple steps needed to go gluten free! If you experience any problem while following these steps you can contact me through my website, www.glutenfreeEm.com, and I will be happy to offer you some advice. I guarantee that if I don't know the answer to your question, I will try my best to steer you in the direction you need to go to find it!

With these simple steps, you can become totally gluten free and begin regaining your health. Do not forget to reread the steps to be sure that you have not overlooked anything. If you are gluten intolerant, the slightest bit of gluten can make you sick so be sure that you are very careful. In addition, do not forget to watch out for cross-contamination (contact with something that has gluten in it can transfer gluten to the gluten free food, for example using the same utensil to dish it with). Even kissing someone who has just eaten something with gluten in it. Just as you would avoid peanuts if you had a peanut allergy, you should avoid gluten if you have a severe sensitivity to eat.

For more information, you can go to my website www.glutenfreeEm.com and find recipes, product recommendations, and helpful links to other websites that offer help with the gluten free diet.

I hope that this information has been a help to you, and I pray it changes your life in a positive way. Have a Happy, Healthy, Gluten Free Day!

~Gluten Free Em~

Please check out my cookbook, "Cooking Gluten and Corn Free with Gluten Free Em" for recipes to help you on this journey of eating gluten free. For signed copies of the cookbook, or this book, please email me at: contactglutenfreeem@gmail.com

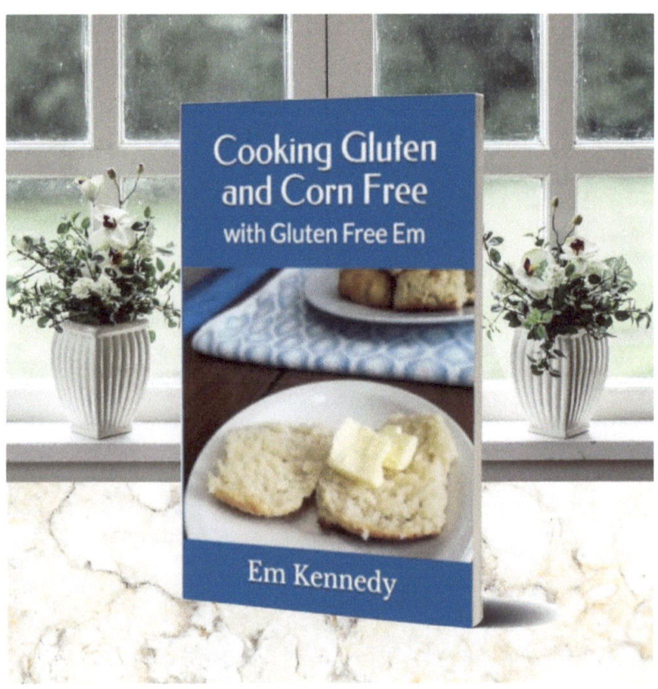

www.ingramcontent.com/pod-product-compliance
Lightning Source LLC
Chambersburg PA
CBHW040305240726
48664CB00006B/1382